Your Loved One Is Coming Home

Ways to Help Prepare Yourself to Take Care of a Loved One During Their Last Days

JOAN LEHRKE

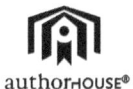

authorHOUSE®

AuthorHouse™
1663 Liberty Drive
Bloomington, IN 47403
www.authorhouse.com
Phone: 1-800-839-8640

First published by AuthorHouse   10/7/2009

ISBN: 978-1-4490-3485-6 (e)
ISBN: 978-1-4490-3484-9 (sc)

Library of Congress Control Number: 2009910222

Printed in the United States of America
Bloomington, Indiana

This book is printed on acid-free paper.

Dedication

This booklet is dedicated to the loved ones I've had in my life. As I get older, it seems as though the moments spent with them are more and more special. Even though there are only a few people listed in this book, there are many others I have been fortunate enough to have had in my life that are gone now. Taking care of Mae and Tom were an opportunity for me to try and "make up" for not having been old enough, mature enough, or close enough in proximity to help with the others I have loved that are no longer with us.

It is my hope that if you are in the position of taking care of a loved one during their last days that you will consider it an honor and be able to do what it necessary out of love and respect. For remember....we all will have our own last days.

Information I Need To Know About My Loved One....

_____

First Name   Middle Name   Last Name

_____   _____

Date of Birth   Place of Birth

_____

Social Security Number

_____

Medicare or Health Insurance Number

_____

Name and Phone Number of Primary Health Insurance Company

Policy and/or Group Number_____

_____

Name and Phone Number of Other Health Insurance Company

Policy and/or Group Number_____

_____   _____

Religion   Place of Worship

_____

Name and Number of Religious Representative to Contact

Your loved one is coming home. Emotions are running high. Perhaps there is a rehabilitation period to go through before he/she is able to get back to normal activity. Possibly there has been a decline and his/her health that causes a change in how "normal" will now be. Or, maybe your loved one has come home to spend the last part of their life and you are fortunate enough to be able to have them with you until the end. Whatever your circumstances, there are going to be some things you will encounter that life may never have thrown your way before. This pamphlet is an attempt to help you through some of these changes.

Before going further I'd like to introduce myself and let you know why writing this pamphlet is so important to me. I am Joan Lehrke, an ordinary person who, until recently, had no real experience with taking care of a dying family member. Yes, I took care of my children all through the ear infections, stitches, and various illnesses, but not until recently did I actually have someone look at me and place their final days in my hands – what a humbling, terrifying, gratifying honor. My mother-in-law, Mae Lehrke, was 87 years old and seemed to be in extremely good health and definitely had all her faculties about her. As a matter of fact, less than a year prior she had taken care of her son-in-law as he lost a very hard fought battle with cancer. Tom (Tommy) Wolf was diagnosed with cancer in July of 2006 and died at home in March 2007. During that time Mae helped Fran (her daughter – Tom's wife) with the entire hospice process. Together Fran and Mae went from the shock of learning the terrible diagnosis to taking care of Tommy through the good days and the bad days, to the emptiness in the house after Tom passed and the visitors stopped coming by.

But then Mae herself was hospitalized with bronchitis. The day after my husband Don and I returned from vacation we received a phone call from one of Don's sisters informing us that Mae was to be admitted into a nursing home to "rehabilitate" from her bronchitis. The doctors said it would take two to three weeks for her to recover.

Doctor to Contact in Case of Questions (Name and Phone Number)

If More Than One Doctor Involved, then Names and Numbers:

_____

_____

_____

_____

Name and Number of Hospice/Visiting Nurse Provider

_____

Name and Phone Number of Visiting Nurse

_____

Name and Number of Nursing Assistant

Without hesitation we made the three-hour trip to pick Mae up and bring her home with us. When we picked her up at the hospital Mae was on oxygen full-time, breathing treatments every four hours, had almost more medications to take than I could keep track of, and was now wearing "Depends" because she would lose control while coughing, and was too weak to make it to the bathroom in time. We had seen Mae just two weeks prior and she was not sick at all then. It was hard to believe this was the same person!

After several days of rest, faithfully administering breathing treatments, medicine, and eating well, Mae appeared to be on the mend. As a matter of fact, when the physical therapist came to visit and prepare an in-home treatment plan, Mae found the strength to walk on her own, lie down on her own, and was even smiling for the therapist. Until then Mae had not been able to walk without great assistance, or lie down without coughing. This was a wonderful day, and the beginning of a string of "worst days" of our lives.

Just the evening prior I had noticed a bruise on Mae's right side that was not there before. I was of the understanding that the visiting nurse would be stopping by and hoped to be able to show it to her. Could it have happened when Mae's daughters and I were helping her out of the bathtub the other day? Could she have lost her balance and fallen against something in the hospital and I wasn't aware until now? She always slept on this side, was she somehow spending too much time (on this one side) during her sleeping hours – how could that be, she was only in bed for sleeping and then up in the chair the rest of the day. I had spoken with the visiting nurse who stated she would not be by, but the physical therapist would be. So, before he left I asked the physical therapist to look at the bruise on Mae's side. The therapist was immediately alarmed and asked if Mae had fallen. Since she had only been with us for 5 days, I could only answer for that time frame and no – she had not. When he lifted Mae's blouse and his eyes widened to my horror I looked and the bruise had grown to the point that it now covered her entire torso on the front to the

Who Should I call?

Family Members to be Contacted:

_____   _____
Name   Phone Number(s)

_____   _____
Name   Phone Number(s)

_____   _____
Name   Phone Number(s)

_____   _____
Name   Phone Number(s)

_____   _____
Name   Phone Number(s)

_____   _____
Name   Phone Number(s)

_____   _____
Name   Phone Number(s)

_____   _____
Name   Phone Number(s)

back. We took Mae to the emergency room and right away they did a CAT scan and discovered she was in stage 4 cirrhosis of the liver, had kidney failure, COPD, and after further tests determined that her bone marrow was no longer "making blood."

From that point things continued to spiral downward. Mae spent several days in the hospital where they were able to stabilize her and sift through the medical files sent from her primary doctor and specialists in the "big city." After a team of 4 local doctors reviewed her tests results and looked her case over with fresh eyes, it was determined that Mae would be passing away…soon.

Of course we were upset and saddened that our time with Mae was now to be ended sooner than any of us thought. No matter how old a person may be, when they have all their senses about them and are a joy to be around, it is a great blow to learn they will no longer be there.

After spending several days in the hospital Mae was released. She was on the oxygen full-time…that would not change. Her medications were adjusted, with most of the old ones being discontinued and just a few added in their place. Mae also had a catheter, so she did not wear "Depends" until she was no longer able to reach the toilet or commode for bowel movements.

The nurses and doctors told us many things to do, mainly to focus on comfort, and not cure; they arranged for the visiting nurse to stop by several times a week; and advised Mae to get her affairs in order. All of these things we needed to hear, and greatly appreciated. But, they could not tell us everything else there was to *know, watch for, and do*.

Although I am an average individual, not in the medical profession, It is my hope that with this pamphlet, written from the experiences of my family, and advice from your loved one's doctor, the visiting nurse, and your minister, priest, etc., you will find the inner strength and confidence to help you and your family through this very delicate time.

Family and Friends to Contact (Continued):

Name   Phone Number(s)

Name   Phone Number(s)

Name   Phone Number(s)

Name   Phone Number(s)

Name   Phone Number(s)

Name   Phone Number(s)

Name   Phone Number(s)

Name   Phone Number(s)

Name   Phone Number(s)

What Items Should We Take With Us
From The Hospital?

What Services are Available to Help Take Care of My Loved One Once He/She is Home? Many hospitals have social workers or patient advocates that help make arrangements with a home hospice company. *Be sure that you are put in contact with this person before your loved one is discharged.* If your loved one is on Medicare, there is a program called "Medicare Hospice" that is so incredibly wonderful you must take advantage of it. Medicare Hospice will cover many, many of the costs incurred in taking care of a loved one in your own home. It will cover everything from the oxygen that they can arrange to be delivered (if necessary), to the visiting nurse, to the certified nursing assistant to the supplies you will need such as, but definitely not limited to: the hospital bed, wheelchair, walker, commode, and even the hospital bedside table.

How Do I Prepare for My Loved One to Come Home? You will need to coordinate with the social worker or patient care coordinator. He/she will make the arrangements for you as to what equipment and medications you need. A doctor's order is needed for the medications, as well as the equipment to be delivered. As far as what particular equipment you may need, you can consult with the social worker or patient care coordinator for what may be necessary items. TRY TO HAVE THE OXYGEN, BED, MATTRESS, COMMODE, AND WHEELCHAIR ALL ARRIVE BEFORE YOUR LOVED ONE GETS HOME FROM THE HOSPITAL. For their own health and your peace of mind it is extremely necessary to have at least the hospital bed and oxygen there before they arrive. This is an emotional, trying time for all and to relieve apprehension and anxiety it is best to have these essentials before you get home with your loved one.

Other Service Providers:

Name of Oxygen Supply Company:

_____

Number(s) for Oxygen Supply Company:

_____

What Setting Has the Doctor Prescribed for the Oxygen to Start?

_____

Be Sure to Tell ALL Visitors that there is NO SMOKING in the House/Apartment Because Oxygen is in Use!!!

Name of Bed and Equipment Supply Company:

_____

Number(s) for Bed and Equipment Supply Company:

_____

What Size Sheets Do You Need for the Bed?   Are the Fitted Sheets also Delivered, or do you need to supply them?

_____

If possible, ask the patient care advocate or social worker to find out if an air mattress is allowable through your loved one's healthcare provider. We found that an air bed lessened Mae's pain in her spine. Not only that, it was much more comfortable for her and seemed to "cradle" her so that she did not slip in the bed quite as much.

Most of the hospital beds used in home settings take twin-size sheets, but ask the patient care advocate to double check so that you can be sure to have a set of sheets on hand when the bed arrives, or shortly afterward.

The oxygen will probably be delivered from a company separate from the one that provides the hospital bed and other equipment. The delivery person will provide you with quick instructions and at first this may seem a little overwhelming, but with a little care and caution you will do just fine. Remember though, as long as the oxygen is in the house there should be NO SMOKING in the house/apartment./

The oxygen delivery company will probably give you several small tanks and one larger unit that "creates" oxygen from the air in your home. It is important to keep the level set at least what the doctor orders. Double-check with your nurse or doctor before leaving the hospital and ask them if it would be OK to turn the oxygen level up a little BEFORE your loved one needs to exert him or herself, and then put the level back down AFTER your loved one has settled in from their exertion. This would mean before getting up to go to the bathroom or commode, before getting up from a chair, before getting out of bed, any time they need to expend more energy than they do in a resting position. I found by raising the oxygen just a little that it helps keep them comfortable. But, ask the doctor or visiting nurse if this is appropriate for your circumstances.

Meeting with the Doctor/Team of Healthcare Providers:

Did you and your family have an opportunity to meet with the Doctor and the team of Healthcare providers?

What Was Determined to Be the Prognosis?

_____

_____

_____

Did the Doctor Give Any Indication as to What to Watch For/Do?

_____

_____

_____

_____

_____

Before Leaving the Hospital

Before leaving the hospital be sure that you ask for a meeting with the team that cared for your loved one (doctors for each specialty involved, as well as the social worker and/or patient advocate) and the immediate family. The doctors may or may not offer for your loved one to be present during this meeting. Or, they may suggest that the immediate family meet first without your loved one present and then invite your loved one to attend after the family members have had an opportunity to absorb not only the enormity of the situation, but the fact that there are care giving responsibilities to be handled that possibly no one in the family has ever had exposure to before. During this meeting ask the doctor(s) to be as blunt and down to earth as possible. This opportunity to speak with your loved one's doctor(s) needs to be used to its fullest so that all involved understand the prognosis, what has caused the diagnosis they have come up with, and what symptoms you as caregivers should look for. Ask point blank if your loved one need continue or receive blood transfusions (in Mae's case it made no sense for her to continue transfusions, as they would no longer be effective and transporting her to and from the facility would be more taxing for her physical wellbeing than would be useful.) Ask if your loved one needs to continue on the same medication as they have in the past, or if there is a medication change (either in dosage or in prescription). Also, be sure to get a business card from each of the doctor(s), social workers, and/or patient care advocates that attend.

It is extremely important that family members understand the prognosis. If your loved one will be not recovering, then the focus will be on keeping your loved one as comfortable as possible. This sounds very simple, very logical, and straightforward, but once the different personalities and perspectives are brought into place, there can be differences of opinions.

Please remember that everyone loves your loved one in their own way, but each person involved may have an idea of what needs to be done.

Do You, as a Caregiver, Have a Copy of Your Loved One's Directive (or other document on file with the doctor and hospital)?

This document states whether or not your loved one would like to be put on life support (if the situation arises) and who can make health care arrangements in the event he or she is unable to do so.

Who is the person(s) that will be making care decisions on behalf of your loved one?

_____   _____
Name   Phone Number(s)

_____   _____
Name   Phone Number(s)

If you are not the person assigned to make the care giving decisions, then be sure to keep the person(s) assigned to do so updated on a frequent and regular basis as to how your loved one is doing.

Sometimes it can be very difficult for a family member to understand that in one's last days it is not necessarily important to be sure what is eaten is "healthy". By forcing your loved one to eat, exercise, or even to carry on conversations when they do not want to, this is not allowing them to be comfortable. If your loved one wants chocolate cake for breakfast and ice cream for lunch, followed by pudding for dinner, then let them have it. (Please know that this is the advice I received during Mae's last days.) At this stage of the game there is no need to worry about eating something that will cause their cholesterol level to rise, or to force them to eat their vegetables because it is "good for them." Remember, these are your loved one's last days and what they crave for food may not be what you agree with, but it is still your loved one's last days and their comfort is what is of the most importance. If they ask for something that gives them intestinal distress, or does not "sit well" with them, then suggest something else, but leave their wants up to them and see what you can do to accommodate. As the days go on you will find that he or she will want less to eat and eventually it may come to where Jell-O or popsicles are the bulk of their menu.

DNR (Do Not Resuscitate) Bracelet - Discuss with your loved one whether or not they want to have CPR performed on them, when they stop breathing, etc. If they do not want anyone to try to prolong their life, then be sure to get a DNR (Do Not Resuscitate) bracelet and have your loved one wear it. This is to prevent medical personnel from having to perform mandatory CPR – when, in fact, that is the last thing your loved one wants. As of this date, the State of Wisconsin requires that all medical personnel perform lifesaving procedures on all patients that have stopped breathing…unless they have a DNR bracelet. There are only two types of bracelets honored by the State of Wisconsin in this situation and both of them require a doctor's signature. So please, be sure to get the proper bracelet from your physician before your loved one is released from the hospital. (In the state of Wisconsin the proper bracelet is not on the wrist of the patient, then emergency personnel are required by law to perform lifesaving maneuvers, even if it is the explicit wish of the patient and loved

Medications:

Name of Medicine	Dosage	Frequency/Time of Day:
_____	_____	_____
_____	_____	_____
_____	_____	_____
_____	_____	_____
_____	_____	_____
_____	_____	_____
_____	_____	_____
_____	_____	_____
_____	_____	_____
_____	_____	_____
_____	_____	_____
_____	_____	_____
_____	_____	_____
_____	_____	_____

one that no medical procedures be performed.) Performing resuscitation does not come without risk to the patient, so please be sure if it is your loved one's wish not to be resuscitated, then the proper bracelet is worn.

How Do I Get My Loved One Home? If you are unable to take your loved one home in your own vehicle for various reasons (i.e. you do not own a vehicle, you have a truck or some other type of vehicle that requires more help from your loved one than they are able to give, or you are just not sure you can do this on your own) there are services available where the social worker or patient care advocate is able to make arrangements for a van with a lift to give your loved one a ride to your home. Although you must remember there is a charge for this service, we found it to be an absolute Godsend. The gentleman that drove the van was so wonderful, he was thoughtful to be sure Mae was warm enough (March in Wisconsin is still cold), he was attentive to Mae during the trip in talking with her and putting on music that she liked, and when we got to our home he was able to help us bring her up the stairs – we lived in a bi-level so no matter which way we went there were stairs. I joined Mae in the van for the ride, but just sat there while she enjoyed looking out the windows and getting outside for what was to be her last time.

Medications at Home - As far as medication goes when you arrive at home, the visiting nurse will monitor the medications you may be giving your loved one. As time goes by there may be some medications that are discontinued or decreased (or maybe increased). When your loved one gets closer to their last days a painkiller will quite possibly be prescribed. At first I was very concerned that possibly I would give Mae too much, -- one day she took a nap that lasted nearly 24 hours! That scared me and I thought possibly she was leaving us sooner than anyone had warned, but she woke up, visited with everyone, ate a little, and was perfectly fine. However, during her nap it was very scary for

What other family member(s) and friends can fill in for you during caregiving to give you a break in order to take care of things, or give you time away?

Name _____   Number _____

Days of the Week or Hours They Can Come Over _____

Name _____   Number _____

Days of the Week or Hours They Can Come Over _____

Name _____   Number _____

Days of the Week or Hours They Can Come Over _____

Name _____   Number _____

Days of the Week or Hours They Can Come Over _____

all of us. This nap seemed to do wonders for Mae because she woke up and wanted to speak with the family and let everyone know what personal items she wished each family member to have and talked about old times with each person that visited. It was a wonderful day, as Mae was the center of attention and stories of old times were told; there were tears of joy and tear of sadness, but everyone there had an opportunity to tell Mae how much they loved her. Less than two weeks later, Mae passed on. But I digress.

The medication should not be withheld because you are concerned that your loved one will become dependent, or that you just are not quite certain that your loved one is in "enough" pain to warrant a pain killer. Remember, some of the painkillers also make it easier for the lungs to function and for your loved one to breathe and, it is easier to take care of pain as it arises than it is to chase down pain and try to get it under control. When in doubt, contact your visiting nurse.

Going from Cure to Comfort

In the case of your loved one coming home to rehabilitate, then you will be doing all possible to help them during the rehabilitation process, whether it be having therapists and/or nurses come to your home, or transport your loved one to the facility required in order for them to travel their road to wellness.

However, many of us will be bringing our loved one home for their last days. Not only is it emotionally hard to adjust to the idea that they will not be "getting better," but there are other considerations that fall into place.

Other Resources to Help Us Through This Time:
(Books, Videos, Audio Tapes, etc.)

_____

_____

_____

_____

_____

_____

_____

_____

_____

_____

_____

_____

_____

_____

Prepare Yourself for the Phases – The hospital may offer to you a pamphlet that will help guide you through the different phases your loved one will go through. Please, take and read this pamphlet. No one person follows all the phases exactly as any one book has written, but there are certain things every person will go through in their last days and it helps as their caregiver to know what to watch for. The hospital gave us a pamphlet entitled: Gone From My Sight – The Dying Experience, written by Barbara Karnes. This pamphlet became very important to the entire family during both Mae's and Uncle Tom's last days.

Be Ready to Write

At the hospital you probably took many notes as to what the doctors diagnosed, what the prognosis may be, and the signs and symptoms you were given to be watchful for. Keep these notes, as you may need to refresh your mind later. At the hospital when you are given all this information, it may not all register, as this is surely a trying time and your mind and emotions are probably sent in a tailspin.

Not only will you need to write down directions from the doctor, visiting nurse, and other caregivers involved, you should write down the times and amounts of each medication you administer to your loved one. This may sound like a "no brainer," but there will be times you get so busy, that you may not remember exactly when, or exactly how much pain medication, or other type of medication, you needed to administer.

Also, write down things like what time your loved one took a nap, fell asleep for the evening, had a meal, had a bowel movement, etc. This information will come in handy later when the visiting nurse, doctor, or other provider needs to know.

Tips Given by Others to Help Make Caregiving Easier:

(There may be other family or friends that have been through the care giving experience and have suggestions to offer. Please do not discount this advice – some will work for you and some will not, but try to write down what they offer.)

_____

_____

_____

_____

_____

_____

_____

_____

_____

_____

_____

_____

_____

_____

_____

Oxygen - Once your loved one has arrived home, there will be a flurry of activity on your part to be sure they are comfortable, have been hooked up to the oxygen (if needed), have their medication (if needed), and you have your bearings. If you have turned the oxygen up before they exerted themselves for the move home, then remember to turn it back to what your doctor has prescribed as a "normal" level.

Water in the Oxygen to Alleviate Dry Nose – Dry nose from oxygen is hard to avoid. This is uncomfortable, so ask about turning on the water canister before his or her nose gets dry. Not only can this cause a dry nose, but sometimes a little bleeding, so be watchful.

Cutting the Garment Up the Back – We found that for a woman once she is no longer able to easily assist in getting dressed and undressed, it makes sense to have them wear a nightgown with a zipper down the front. This works quite well from a caregiving aspect, but as their ability to move lessens, it will help to cut the nightgown all the way up the center of the back. By doing so you can remove the garment even more easily when needed to either get it out of the way to clean up messes, give sponge baths, or change to a clean nightgown. These can usually be found in the women's section of a department store in the pajama area.

For a man, simply cut a t-shirt up the back and let it lay open in the back, but covering the front. When it comes to his bottoms, definitely nothing requiring a zipper or button closure – for a while a pair of lounge pants or pajama bottoms that can be easily slipped up and down will work. Later it may be necessary to switch to adult diapers (Depends is an example). If that is the case, you may try one "Depends" left open on the bottom (not affixed by the tab strip) and one "Depends" left open on top.

Definitely do not put them in anything that needs to go over the head because you are just asking for inconvenience, exasperation by doing so. Even worse, you could accidentally hurt them!

More Tips and Advice
(The Visiting Nurse and CAN's are great sources of good advice)

_____

_____

_____

_____

_____

_____

_____

_____

_____

_____

_____

_____

_____

_____

_____

_____

If There is a Catheter – You will always need to be watchful of the tube. But, we found that the catheter made things so much easier. Not only was there less cleanup, but less chance for irritation on the skin from urine. Ultimately it is up to your loved one whether or not he or she wants a catheter. Catheters do requiring a little cleaning around the area, but a nurse can tell you what to do. In our state only the nurse or visiting nurse can insert a catheter, if it is not inserted at the hospital, you can request one later on if necessary.

The Gait Belt – When we left the hospital, one of my husband's sisters came home with a gait belt. If the hospital does not give you one, which they probably will not, then you will need to purchase one from a hospital supply store. I do not know how expensive they are, but they can turn out to be invaluable. Ask the nurses to show you how to use this belt. This belt, when properly placed around your loved one, will assist you in getting your loved one lifted out of bed, lifted off of the commode, and give you something to hold onto when walking them from one location to another (no matter how short the distance). It is my suggestion that after your loved one is feeling too tired or weak to manage without assistance (or even before that time) you use the gait belt. We got to the point where we did not remove the belt while using the commode, even though it was right next to the bed, because it made no sense to keep putting it on and taking it off. Either after they sit back on the side of the bed, or after they are lying down you can take the belt back off again. Talk to the nurse or visiting nurse and ask them more about the gait belt.

Things My Loved One Likes now and Dislikes now:

(Example: food, music, television program, smells – such as perfumes and soaps, topics of discussion, etc.)

LIKES:

_____

_____

_____

_____

_____

_____

DISLIKES:

_____

_____

_____

_____

_____

_____

Likes and dislikes may change

It is sometimes hard to get used to the idea that things our loved one used to enjoy eating may not appeal to them anymore. Also, the reverse seems to happen in that things you never saw them eat before they suddenly crave. There may have been studies done as to why this happens, but all I can advise is that if you notice this to be the case, do not be alarmed, just get them what they would like, and laugh about the change. Maybe it is just as simple as there are things he/she have always wanted to try and never have, so this is probably their last chance to try whatever food item it is.

I even noticed with my Uncle Tom, whom I helped hospice one week after Mae passed, how likes change. During Mae's last couple of weeks she really enjoyed having her feet and legs rubbed with lotion. It was the massage that she liked more than the lotion, but it made her feel comfortable. Well, shortly after arriving at Aunt Arlene and Uncle Tom's, I placed a footstool in front of Uncle Tom's chair, propped one of his feet up on my lap and started to massage his foot (with the socks on). Aunt Arlene walked into the room, her eyes got huge, and her mouth fell open. She couldn't believe that he allowed me to rub his feet. Uncle Tom had been a diabetic for many years and he was very protective of his feet, and on several occasions Aunt Arlene had offered to massage his feet for him, but he'd always said "no" and wouldn't allow her to do so. So, after Aunt Arlene explained her surprise to me, I asked Uncle Tom if he would like me to continue rubbing his feet, or should I leave them alone. His reply was to lean the recliner back and put both feet on my lap. But, this little revelation was actually one of the best things that could've happened for my aunt and uncle. For the rest of his time at home before he passed, which was only a week, Aunt Arlene would sit down in front of Uncle Tom, gently rub his feet and do what I refer to as "just be". That means sitting quietly, not forcing conversation, and touching each other to let each other know they are loved.

Sizes

(Sizes of garments/adult disposables, slippers, etc.)

Size and brand of adult disposable needed

_____

Size of t-shirt or blouse:

_____

Size of pants (if worn):

_____

Size of nightgown:

_____

Size of Slippers:

_____

Other Sizes for Items not Mentioned Above:

_____

_____

_____

_____

Put a Plastic Bag in the Commode – As we all know, when a person has a bowel movement, the quality of aroma in the air can change, and not for the good. You will be busy wiping your loved one (with moist towlettes) after the bowel movement and there is no water to flush the commode next to the bed…So, I suggest placing a plastic bag inside the commode and then tossed the used towlettes into the commode to all be tied up in the bag and disposed of as soon as your loved one is tucked comfortably back into bed. If there is just urine in the bag, then the bag can be dumped into the toilet and then disposed of. If there is anything else in the bag, then tie it up and get it to the dumpster as soon as possible.

Adult Disposables - Let them know that it is OK to go to the bathroom in their Depends. That means both urination, and bowel movement. There will come a time when it is just too dangerous to have them get up to use the commode. However, until then, if they are comfortable, place the commode in the room so that you can easily grab it and put it near the bed for easier use. As I stated before, line the commode with a plastic bag and clean up will be much easier.

Feeling Fresh (Tooth/Denture Brushing, Mouth Swish) – Let's face it, all of us, whether we wear dentures or not, need to have our teeth brushed in order to maintain a sense of freshness, and not become offensive to others in close proximity. Until your loved one is no longer eating and is sleeping almost all the time, they may appreciate being freshened up with the opportunity to have their teeth brushed. If they wear dentures, then take out the dentures, clean them, and don't forget to still brush the inside of the mouth. If he or she would like, then even a swish of mouthwash works well when brushing doesn't seem an option anymore.

Things Noticed That I'd Like to Ask the Visiting Nurse or Doctor About:

(example: sore or "blemish" that was not there before)

_____

_____

_____

_____

_____

_____

_____

_____

_____

_____

_____

_____

_____

A Little Spritz can Make a Big Difference - Spritzing perfume or cologne on bed sheets (or for use after the commode) can go a long way to help feeling fresh…but don't overdue it. Remember, if he or she is already having trouble breathing, then don't overpower them with scent.

Gently Rub Their Feet and Legs – Make the offer to rub lotion on their feet and legs (even their arms and face if they'd like). Not only does this make them feel better, but it gives you an opportunity to look for any bedsores or tissue breakdown.

Bedsores and Tissue Breakdown – This will probably occur. If you are lucky, it will not, but do not be surprised. Bedsores happen when a person is lying in one position for a period of time. There is a cream (referred to as "barrier cream") the visiting nurse will give to you to apply to these sores – don't be afraid to use it. Bedsores can become infected very easily, so please show the visiting nurse any sores that you notice.

Tissue breakdown may also occur. We were instructed to keep the legs elevated on a pillow and not let the feet press against the footboard of the bed. This can be hard to accomplish, but every time you go into the room you should take a "peek" at their feet and be sure they are not pressing on the footboard. Also, some people like to cross their ankles, creating pressure points for the tissue to breakdown. If this is the case, then ask the visiting nurse about padded booties made especially for keeping the pressure off these points as much as possible.

No Wrinkles in the Sheets – Avoid having the sheets "bunch" up under your loved one. These wrinkles can also add to bedsores. Whatever you do, though, please be gentle in pulling the wrinkles out of the sheets. The skin has a tendency to become very fragile, and you do not want to cause any more undue discomfort, or sores.

Use a Baby Monitor – A monitor can be a great tool to allow you to step away; your loved one needs privacy when they want, and so do you. Taking the monitor from room to room will allow you to hear if you are called for, or if there is a change in breathing that requires an adjustment in oxygen, or anything else you may need to hear. But, when visitors were in the room we were sure to shut the monitor off in order to give our loved one and the visitors privacy.

Moving Your Loved One in the Bed - When moving your loved one back up the bed, because they will have a tendency to slide down (try to do so with a helper and then hook your arms under their armpits and both lift at the same time) or ask the visiting nurse for other ways in which to accomplish this task. Once your loved one is no longer able to be "lifted" in this way, you should get someone to help you. We took a sheet, separate folded it, and laid it on top of the bottom sheet so that we could use it as a "lifter". This "lifter" went from mid-thigh to above the shoulder area. When it came time to raise back toward the top of the bed, we would count 1-2-3 and then both lift at the same time using the "lifter" sheet. This way there is no effort needed by your loved one, no skin is damaged, and with two people things go much easier. REMEMBER: ASK THE VISITING NURSE FOR TIPS ON HOW TO DO SOME OF THESE THINGS. There can also be hospice people available to come several times a day or week to help you with these tasks.

Dry Mouth and Dry Lips – This becomes a bigger problem as time progresses and your loved one drinks less fluid. Use a swab dunked in water to hydrate and rinse the inside of the mouth. And, use lip balm/ Vaseline on their lips. This is another area where it helps to start before his or her lips are dry, so maybe make it a habit right away to several times a day "hydrate" their lips. Even with vigilance, they could still end up with dry/chapped lips, but do your best.

Let's Just Pretend - Sometimes you may need to pretend. Yes, my Uncle Tom felt very strongly that the article he thought he had on his lap be placed on the bookshelf. There was nothing in his hands, or on his lap, but until I let him think I was taking the article away and placing it where he wanted on the shelf, he would not calm down. So, there may be times when you need to act as though you are doing something in order to help them stay calm.

Playing "Possum" As hard as it may be to believe, your loved one may decide to play "possum" and pretend to be asleep. We found this almost incomprehensible, but it did happen. Mae explained that she just didn't have the mental energy to talk to some of the people around, and she did not want to hurt their feelings, so she pretended to be asleep. That was fine with us because we knew she was such a lady that she would never want to hurt anyone's feelings, but yet at the same time she needed her space and time to herself.

Who is He/She Talking To? – Your loved one may "talk" in their sleep to others that have already passed on. We found this to be the case, but when we asked afterward, our loved one did not remember the experience. So, this may or may not happen in your instance, but know that it can.

Extremely Emotional Visitors – In my opinion…DON'T LET THEM IN UNTIL THEY HAVE COMPOSED THEMSELVES. Yes, there will be tears, but your loved one does not need the added stress of someone who is uncontrollable or hysterical coming into their room and "unloading" or making a scene. Remember…this is the time for your loved one – not the time for the hysterical visitor.

Arrangements That Need to be Dealt With:

Any particulars your loved one or family would like mentioned in the obituary:

_____

_____

_____

_____

Funeral Home Name and Number:

_____

Funeral Home Contact Person and Location:

_____

Do you have a particular Florist in Mind, or Do You Prefer the Funeral Home Make a Recommendation:

_____

Any Certain Flowers or Colors?

Do You Have All the Paperwork Necessary for Special Arrangements, such as Military Services, etc?

If Your Family is Making a Memory Board(s), or CD for the services? If so, then the items should be gotten together.

Funeral/Memorial Arrangements – Let's face it; these arrangements need to be dealt with. The sooner you involve the funeral home, the better. Maybe you have quite a while before you will actually need their services, maybe not. In any event, ask your loved one what their wishes are. It is not unheard of for the person passing to want to have a great deal of input regarding their services.

Meeting with the funeral home representatives will not only give you an idea of the cost financially, but the alternatives available for cremation/ burial/caskets, when and how to arrange for specific music, who may be available from the different religious denominations to preside over the service, how would you like the obituary to read, and perhaps there are individuals that may speak their remembrances during the service. Possibly your loved one belonged to the armed forces, or special organization that they would like to have involved in the service. If your loved one is the spouse of someone buried in a veteran's cemetery and they would like to be buried alongside their deceased husband or wife, then you will need to make arrangements with the cemetery, and there is additional paperwork involved – so find out what is needed and try to find out from your loved one where the information is kept – if possible. Also, many times a meal is served after the service; the decision will need to be made as to where the meal will be, what it will be, and how it will be paid for.

Be sure to ask the funeral home representatives what they need from you the day they come to pick your loved one up from your home (or wherever they may be) and take them to the funeral home. Ask all the questions you can think of. I know of one young whose father was hospiced at home. Once the father had passed, the young man insisted that the father be dressed in the clothes he was to be buried in <u>before</u> being taken from the home. This young man was devastated when he learned that there was just no way it was feasible to fulfill such a request. Had he asked, or stated this was his wish ahead of time, then the family would've been saved the added emotional upset of the young man refusing to allow his father's body to be released until the funeral director

If Your Loved One Has Not Had the Opportunity to Their Goodbyes to Anyone, is There Something They Want Known to That Person for You to Pass Along?

_____

_____

_____

_____

_____

_____

_____

_____

_____

_____

_____

could calm him down and explain the process the funeral home must undergo prior to the body being "laid out." So, please, talk over your wishes with your loved one, and your funeral home representative.

The Death Certificate – This document is usually not thought of during the course of most of our days. However, the person or people handling the affairs on behalf of your loved one after they are gone will need this document. I believe it was the funeral director that asked how many copies we needed and ordered them to be sent via the mail to one of us. (We ordered at least one for each of the adult children and an extra two or three for the executor.) There may be credit card accounts, other bank accounts, etc. that require a certified copy of the death certificate in order for final business to be conducted on behalf of your loved one after they are gone.

Some of the other lessons I learned were:

Let others help. You should not be alone in this. If you take on 100% of the caregiving, you are not doing justice to yourself of your loved one. Yes, be there....yes, keep an ear out and eyes open, but if at all possible Do Not Do It All Yourself. You will wear yourself out physically (and then be of less use to yourself, your loved one, and your family) and you will wear yourself out emotionally (which can be worse than physically).

Let others feel needed. If they want to help by making meals, doing laundry, reading a book out loud to your loved one, watching television together, passing time just being together or taking a shift for sitting up...then let them. Remember, this is about your loved one more than about you, and these people are part of your loved one's life. Don't be selfish, but also do take your fair share of the responsibility.

Leave the house once and a while. Go grocery shopping, take a walk, or go for a short drive. Weather permitting, just try to get out of the house for a while. Not only will the break be good for you, you will come back feeling more refreshed, which will, believe it or not, help your loved one to not feel as though they have become a burden.

If family members or friends are not available to sit with your loved one while you are gone, then hospice offers this service. Your loved one does not need to be alone while you step away for a while.

If you have found this pamphlet to be helpful, then it has served its purpose. Should you have any suggestions for change or input, these would be welcome. I can be reached at: Joan Lehrke P.O. Box 204, Almond, WI 54909.

Thank you very much for reading this pamphlet and hopefully you will be more confident and informed when your loved one comes home.

About the Author

Joan and her husband Don spend their time in central Wisconsin on their farm. There they have found that they truly enjoy caring for the animals and living in the country. Having spent the majority of their lives living in larger cities, they have fully embraced their new life.

Joan is a mother of two, stepmother of two and grandmother. She considers herself very fortunate to have the love and encouragement of her family to write this book in order to help others.

After spending most of her career as an administrative assistant in the private, non-profit, and public sectors, Joan made the transition to self-employed in the family business with her husband and sons.

On any given day she can be found taking care of the family business, writing, or milking goats on the farm with her husband.

www.ingramcontent.com/pod-product-compliance
Lightning Source LLC
Chambersburg PA
CBHW050345290526
45785CB00006B/2648